Zema

MW00936396

The New Food Culture

Zema Love Fire

ISBN- 13: 978-1533258236
ISBN-10: 1533258236

Cover Design by: Dan Moore Sr./Brittany Jones

You are your own best thing. The art of evolving and change must start within. Food plays a huge role in your healing process because, it affects our physical wellbeing that must be in balance with our spiritual wellbeing. One cannot evolve into the highest version of your human experience without balancing the two.

~ Zema Love Fire

Acknowledgements

This book is dedicated to the Highest Spiritual Entities of Light that are responsible for my being here and doing this sacred work. I would like to acknowledge my Mother Gail, my Father Lonnie and his wife Wanda, my Grandmother Miss Thelma, my Sister's Cathy and Carlethia, my Nieces Jamison and Carsyn, my Nephews Tj and Cameron, my aunts, my uncles, my cousins, and extended family, and a host of friends and acquaintances, and a very warm thank you to my mentor Mr. Dan Moore Sr. and Brittany Jones and The APEX Museum staff for all of the assistance, support and encouragement, you helped me to find my foundation. And to the Atlanta, Ga. Community and abroad for all of your support. I really appreciate everyone who supported me in all of my healing modalities, to my Ancestors, for orchestrating a remarkable change of events to support the circumstances necessary to achieve my goals and dreams. And, I honor my own spirit, for being still and focused enough to answer the call and translate what was on my Spirit onto paper for the world to see. Ase'

Why I wrote this Book
Introduction

I am a Food Researcher, Natural Living Advocate, Healer, Teacher, Rites of Passage Facilitator, Vegan Chef, and Earth Keeper. After years of research and a host of wisdom invoking life experiences, I realized the need for a book that broke down in "layman" terms what is happening with the Industrial Food Industry, and how to navigate it for better health and wellness. I wanted to share the basics in hopes that it will become a catalyst for those searching for such a spark! If you use this guide, I have no doubt in my mind that it will help you make better choices to create healthier options for yourself, family, and community. This book is also a decoder of sorts because; through my research I ran into so many dead ends that I became overwhelmed with the inconsistent information. But, then I realized that this was on purpose! Anything that challenges the "status quo" and can affect not only profit but, the cultural conditionings planned out for us is considered a threat. This is something that must be protected by legalizing lies and utilizing legal loop holes to keep our health at bay, and our illness at the forefront. Healthy people don't render as high a profit as the sick. They want you to turn the other cheek and believe that your food industry would never betray your trust. They want you to buy into the expensive and creative ad campaigns, and the celebrities that they pay millions to endorse their food products to trick and confuse you. It's all designed to gain your trust and dollars. But, you're deserving of the TRUTH! And, my life's purpose is about seeking out and exposing the truth! I'm worth that, and so is everyone else. We have nothing if we don't have our life. And, the quality of our life is based on the quality of our health. Pay no never mind to the money! It does not take an abundance of money to enjoy healthy meals. I want you to acknowledge that millionaires and billionaires suffer and parish from the same cancer's, and illnesses as the lower income communities. Good health is created, and not bought! If you don't discipline yourself, the recourse can be devastating. NOW is the time, to find our way back to natural and simple! So, let's get started.

Contents

The Inflammation Situation

Those aches and pains are saying things!

What is Inflammation?

Redness, swelling, pain, tenderness, heat, and disturbed function of an area of the body, especially as a reaction of tissues to injurious agents, can be external or internal.

The truth is, we are consuming a lot of chemicals masquerading as food. Many things you currently consider to be "foods" are not. Instead, these items are processed, adulterated, refined, diluted, sweetened, salted, or changed in some way. Unfortunately, most "brand" name foods are not real food anymore because the ingredients have been processed for a long shelf life, which means that most of its beneficial anti-inflammatory components have been lost and salt, sugar, and bad fats and preservatives have been added. These chemicals react with our body's delicate systems causing disease. Aside from the chemicals, there are also some foods that also cause inflammation; mainly due to the cellular food engineering resulting in Genetically Modified Foods (GMO's). There are two types of inflammation; acute inflammation, and chronic inflammation.

Acute Inflammation is a brief inflammatory response to an injury or illness that only lasts a few days. A few examples are injury (twisted ankle, broken bones), bacterial or viral infections, sunburn, and cuts.

Chronic inflammation is when things go south. Inflammation becomes chronic when it stops being an acute response and remains a constant low-level physiological response. Chronic inflammation is when your body no longer has the ability to turn off the inflammation and it starts damaging healthy tissue in your body. It could damage the intestinal lining in your gut and cause digestive problems, it could damage the arteries in your heart and cause heart disease, cancer, Alzheimer's, acne, asthma, irritable bowel syndrome, fibromyalgia or it could damage your joints and cause rheumatoid arthritis. At this point you've created a pro-inflammatory monster.

Inflammation Causing Foods
Sugar, agave, soy, meat, dairy, refined grains (breads, pasta, cereal, pizza) banana's, oranges, mangoes, pineapples, oils (corn, canola, soy), iodized salt, wheat, gluten, alcohol, soda, margarine, lard and coffee.

Inflammation Causing Chemicals
food additives (high fructose corn syrup, monosodium glutamate (MSG), artificial colors, artificial flavoring, aspartame, astaxanthin, benzoic acid/sodium benzoate, BHA/BHT, canthaxanthin, emulsifiers, olestra, partially-hydrogenated oils, potassium bromate, sodium nitrate/nitrate, monoglycerides and diglycerides.

Inflammation FIGHTING Foods

Tomatoes, green leafy vegetables (spinach, kale, collards, mustard greens, dandelion greens, chard, bok choy, and callaloo greens), nuts (almonds, walnuts) fatty fish (wild caught salmon, mackerel, tuna, sardines), strawberries, blueberries, cherries, oranges, raisins, ginger, sweet potatoes, whole grains (brown rice, wild rice, whole oats, quinoa, amaranth, barley, bulgur, millet, spelt), celery, beets, broccoli, coconut oil, chia seeds, flax seeds, aloe vera, shitake mushrooms, and watercress.

Inflammation FIGHTING Herbs

Turmeric, cloves, cinnamon, Jamaican allspice, apple pie spice mix, oregano, Pumpkin pie spice, marjoram, sage, rosemary, thyme, macha tea, tulsi tea, Cayenne, basil, black cohosh, cat's claw, chamomile, cilantro, coriander, Fever few, fo-ti root, ginkgo baloba, gotu kola, hemp, juniper, licorice root, Marshmallow, milk thistle, mint, nettle, nutmeg, psyllium husk, raspberry leaf, Rose hip tea, sarsaparilla, ginseng, slippery elm, soursop, yarrow, uva ursi, Himalayan pink salt, and wild yam.

Did you know???

According to Chinese/Kemetic Energy Medicine
inflammation is a hot/dry condition or "yin
deficiency" meaning your energy flow is out of
balance. Yin representing feminine energy and
yang representing masculine energy. Energy
medicine is not that well known in the western
world because, the American Medical
Association chooses not to embrace this ancient
method of healing.

Mucus Don't Lie

Mucus is a natural jelly like substance that is produced in the nasal passages to lubricate the sinuses, nasal passages, and throat. Your body primarily uses mucus to protect and lubricate your delicate tissues and organs. Mucus is also used to reduce damage that might be caused by: stomach acid, bacteria, viruses, fungi, and other potentially harmful fluids or irritants. When your body is fighting off an intruder of some sort it sends mucus to flush out and protect. When you catch a viral or bacterial infection or have allergies, you produce more mucus when your body over produces it, that is an indicator of acute inflammation in the body as well. When you produce too low amounts of mucus, you experience dry sinuses, dry scratchy throat and eyes, along with a possible dry cough. When mucus is out of normal range, it can come out of the skin as plaque mucus or "psoriasis". It's been proven in numerous tests that people removing dairy and chemicals from their diet saw a sizable improvement or cured their psoriasis all together. Constipation and diarrhea are both indicators of mucus imbalance as well.

Water Facts...

Dr. Masaru Emoto a Japanese doctor of Alternative Medicine is celebrated for discovering that water responds to vibrational energy. Water exposed to positive music creates beautiful crystals, while negative music creates malformed crystals when viewed under a powerful telescope.

The New Way of the Water

The water game has changed!

Did you know that there are different types of water to be used for different reasons? The water game has entered into a new era and all water is not created equal! So, now let's explore the world of water.

Tap Water

Tap water is by far the worst on the list. Our municipal water companies are NOT doing a good job of providing fresh "clean" untainted water. Tap water is treated with a plethora of chemicals! It actually blows my mind that our water is FULL of indigestible chemicals, solvents, and deodorizers. Let's delve into what these chemicals are in greater detail.

Fluoride (sodium fluoride)

To start, I want to tell you that I am also a Certified Dental Asst since 2001. It is taught that fluoride helps promote healthier and stronger teeth, therefore a lot of fluoridated toothpastes, mouthwash, and our municipal water supply have added fluoride. As a former worker of the dental field, I can tell you it's all propaganda! Fluoride is actually a highly toxic substance. Consider the "do not swallow" poison warning that The FDA now requires on all fluoridated toothpaste sold in the U.S. Fluoride is more toxic than lead, but slightly less toxic than arsenic. What's interesting to note is that most developed countries including Japan and **97% of the western European populations do NOT consume fluoridated water. In The U.S., about 70% of the public water supplies is fluoridated. Fluoride is the Only chemical added to water for the purpose of medical treatment.** The U.S. Food and Drug administration (FDA) classifies fluoride as a drug when used to prevent or mitigate disease. Conformed consent is standard practice for all medication, and one of the reasons why most of Western Europe has ruled against fluoridation. Governments force people to take medicine irrespective of their consent. Individual doctors cannot do this to individual patients. The other fact is; the dose cannot be controlled. Once fluoride is put in the water it is impossible to control the dose each individual receives because people drink different amounts of water. Being able to control the dose a patient receives is critical. Swallowing fluoride provides NO benefit. Fluoride is a topical and not systemic. The Centers for Disease Control and Prevention (CDC) in 1999, 2001 acknowledged that fluoride benefits are mainly topical, not systemic. There is no need whatsoever, therefore, to swallow fluoride to protect teeth. The largest survey ever conducted in the US (over 39,000 children from 84 communities) by the National institute of Dental Research showed "little difference" in tooth decay among children in fluoridated and non-fluoridated communities. **Tooth decay is high in low- income communities that have been fluoridated for years.** Despite some claims, to the contrary, water fluoridation cannot prevent the oral health crises that result from rampant poverty, inadequate nutrition, and lack of access to dental care. There have been numerous reports of severe dental crises in low-income neighborhoods of U.S. cities that have been fluoridated for over 20 years (e.g., Boston, Cincinnati, New York City, and Pittsburgh). Fluoride is NOT an essential nutrient, and no disease, not even tooth decay is caused by "fluoride deficiency". We are forced to be medicated and who knows how fluoride interacts with other medications being taken? Did you know fluoride accumulates in the body? Healthy adult kidneys excrete 50-60% of fluoride ingested each day. The remainder accumulates in the body, largely calcifying tissues such as the bones and pineal gland. Infants and children excrete less fluoride from their kidneys and take up to 80% of ingested fluoride into their bones. The fluoride content in bone steadily increases over a lifetime. No health agency in fluoridated countries is monitoring fluoride exposure or side effects. There has never been a single randomized controlled trial to demonstrate fluoridation's effectiveness or safety. Interestingly enough, the U.S. Food and drug administration (FDA) continues to classify fluoride as an "unapproved new drug". But, yet our government adds fluoride to our water supply without proper testing? So, after all that, one has to ask the question what gives? Here's a list of some of the side effects of fluoride; arthritis, bone fracture, brain effects, bone cancer, cardiovascular disease, diabetes, endocrine disruption, gastrointestinal effects, hypersensitivity, kidney disease, male fertility, pineal gland, skeletal/dental fluorosis, thyroid disease, acute toxicity, lower IQ in children, increased led absorption, muscle disorders, dementia, inactivates 62 enzymes and inhibits more than 100, effects formation of antibodies, genetic disorders and cell death, disrupted immune system, and damaged sperm. I really went in on fluoride because, its usage is dangerous and perhaps a lot of people are suffering health issues unknowingly from consuming this toxic chemical on a daily basis.

What's also alarming is that The Environmental Working Group (EWG) has once again released a report that should grab your attention. After analyzing water samples from 201 municipal water systems from 43 states, (EWG) found chemicals considered "probable human carcinogens" in **every** single water system they tested. So what are some of the other chemicals found in tap water?

MtBE: (methyl-tert-butyl Ether)-A chemical added to fuel to raise octane number; a potential human carcinogen at high doses.

Atrazine: This US herbicide is banned in the European Union, is the most common water contaminant in the US. Astrazine is an endocrine disruptor known to feminize animals, and is linked to numerous reproduction problems, breast and prostate, cancer, and impaired immune function in humans.

Pharmaceutical Drugs: A 2008 report found a multitude of drugs in the drinking water of at least 51 million Americans, including pain relievers, cancer drugs, antidepressants, oral contraceptives, blood pressure, and cholesterol drugs.

Glyphosate (Roundup): This toxic herbicide is a carcinogenic in minute amounts and is linked to more than 20 adverse health effects, including cancer, birth defects, and infertility; unfortunately, glyphosate is turning up in the bloodstreams of people all over the world.

Arsenic: An element used for centuries as a deadly poison.

Dioxin: An organic compound which is known to increase the likelihood of cancer.

DDT: A deadly chemical used as an insecticide. It has been linked to diabetes and cancer.

Perchlorite: This is used as an oxidizer in rocket fuel and explosives. Can cause neurological disorders.

HCB (Hexachlorobenzene): Commonly used as a pesticide, HCB can cause cancer and disrupt the endocrine system and interfere with enzyme activity.

Chlorine: This chemical is used to disinfect, and impede the growth mold, fungus, and bacteria. We are all familiar with it in swimming pools. It's very stripping and harsh to the hair and skin. We actually find higher levels of chlorine in our tap water than is recommended safe for swimming pools. High levels of chlorine have been linked to cancer, especially breast cancer.

Purified Water

Purified water can come from any source, but has been purified to remove any chemicals or contaminates. Types of purification include distillation, deionization, reverse osmosis, and carbon filtration. Like distilled water, it has its advantages and disadvantages, the advantages being that harmful chemicals may be taken out and the disadvantages being that beneficial minerals may be taken out as well.

Distilled Water

Distilled water is a type of purified water. It's water that has gone through a rigorous filtration process to strip it not only of contaminants, and natural minerals as well. This water is best for medical use, poultices, facial masks, small appliances like water urns, and steam irons, because if you use it, you won't have mineral build up that you often get when you use tap water. This water is not necessarily the best water for human consumption, since all of the water's natural, and often beneficial, minerals are absent. It's a sterile water.

Spring Water

This is one of the water types that is bottled the most. It's usually from an underground source and may or may not have been treated and purified. Spring water is also the choice that still has its "natural" mineral content. Some waters are completely stripped of everything like distilled water but, then they add man made minerals that may not always assimilate well in the body like calcium chloride, magnesium chloride, and potassium bicarbonate.

Artesian Water

Artesian water is water produced from an artesian well. To be an artesian well the water in the aquifer (a subsurface rock unit that holds and transmits water) must be under enough pressure to force it up the well to a level that is higher than the top of the aquifer. Artesian water is another natural water source that carries natural minerals like spring water. This water is usually not treated or purified.

Alkaline Water (pH balanced)

Ok so for starters, let's break down what pH balance means. So, what is it? The potential for hydrogen (pH) balance of our body is measured on a scale of 0 to 14, 7 being neutral, less than 7 being acidic, and greater than 7 being alkaline. The higher the hydrogen concentration, the more acidic a substance will become. You can purchase expensive water system's that will create pH balanced water of 8 to 11 and over. You can also go a more natural route by using lemon or lime juice or even charging in sunlight in a glass jug.

Did you know???

Sea vegetables are high in natural iodine! Iodine supports the thyroid. Add to soups, salads, or make your own sushi rolls! Some seaweeds that are great to start with are, dulse, nori, hijiki, irish moss, and wakame. Also, adding some wakame to your beans while they're cooking will pull the gas out if you are gassy after eating beans.

The GMO Blues
Genetically Modified Organisms

I often tell my student's when I'm teaching my classes' that we are at war! A silent war has been waged against us in the form of food! And to back it up! We now have an ex war chemical company Monsanto who is responsible for the poison Agent Orange used in the Vietnam War from 1967-1971. It was an herbicide made of a powerful mixture of chemicals and defoliants used by U.S military forces during the Vietnam War to eliminate forest coverage for N. Vietnamese and Viet Cong troops, as well as crops that might be used for food. Due to the 19 million gallons poured over Vietnam during that time, both U.S. soldiers and Vietnamese Veterans' suffered neurological damage, intestinal distress, birth defects, skin irregularities, and cancers. And now, they're feeding us??? It's literally that literal! But first, what is a GMO? An organism whose "genome" genes/chromosome genetic material has been altered by the techniques of genetic engineering so that it's DNA contains one or more gene's not normally found there. While in theory it sounds harmless enough, but the problem is, our bodies' do not recognize it as a food, but more as a foreign entity or chemical triggering the immune system and white blood cells creating low grade inflammation that increases over time. It is by definition, no longer a natural food being how nature intended. That cellular change is causing a lot of reactions in people in the form of allergies, inflammation, suppressed immune system, sleep problems, DNA damage, hyperactivity, cancers, digestive issues, obesity and infertility issues. There's a number of independent studies' done on the effects of gmo foods on the human body, animals and our environment. Monsanto is the leading company responsible with blazing a trail for gmo foods to become the main choice for foods in the U.S. Currently, 80% of the crops grown in the U.S. are now gmo crops. The downfall of this is that, the remaining 20% of non-gmo farms is a mixture of organic and traditional conventional farms that are struggling to stay afloat. Monsanto is a company that has a long history starting in about 1901 as a multi-national agrochemical, agricultural, biotechnology company behind Agent Orange, DDT insecticide, Round-up herbicide, NutraSweet, Bovine Growth Hormone, Celebrex arthritis medicine and, you guessed it! Food!!! Food production had been their latest venture that's allowed them to monopolize the food industry! People don't realize in deeper details that, 98% of the fast food restaurants serve GMO foods. To drive my point further, just say you buy a burger combo from one of your favorite fast food restaurants that means the fries, lettuce, tomatoes, mayo, mustard, catsup, beef patty, cheese, french fries, and soda are all GMO foods! All processed and full of chemicals masquerading as food. Our bodies know the difference! With cancer's and food allergies at an all-time high, one has to wonder? Shouldn't we be living longer and healthier? Why are cancer rates at an all-time high? Research shows that 1 in 2 people will be diagnosed with cancer. Who's really benefiting? The sad truth is, capitalism is winning! Truth is, our food industry is NOT, I repeat is NOT in the health business! It's in the money making business! That means longer shelf life that requires preservatives, additives, high amounts of salt, sugar and a slew of chemicals that most of us can't pronounce! In fact, there's a system in place for you that goes like this. Unhealthy foods cause disease, you go to the doctor, the doctor gives you a prescription, if that prescription causes issue you get another, if medication doesn't work, you are recommended for surgery, if surgery fails, you lose your life or quality of life, then thousands more are spent on medical devices or to put you to rest. This is the story of millions of people every year and most people are missing the connection. Cancer is actually an epidemic right now but, cancer is also big business! As the saying goes, good health doesn't generate enough money! Or the other one, there's no money in the cure! It's like a domino effect, one hit leads to another. The other side of it is economic class. GMO foods are always going to be more largely consumed by poorer communities due to low cost. You see, real food cost's more than chemicals. Fresh organic non-GMO foods are the priciest on the market and the least of choice based on education and affordability for the low income communities. There's a larger ratio of GMO fast food restaurants in low income communities' right along with GMO liquor stores where the grains, fruits and sugars used to make alcoholic beverages are also from GMO crops. Understand that 98% of the foods sold in grocery stores in North America are of GMO origin. In the U.S. we are the so called richest economic nation in the world but, we aren't the healthiest or the longest living nation. Makes one ask the question, what do other countries that don't allow GMO crops or fluoridated water know that we don't? But, the funny thing is, the so called third world or smaller countries' had enough sense to do their own private studies on the effects of GMO's and how introducing them into their environment and food supply would affect their health and the health of future generations. Upon their own research countries like Austria, Wales, France, Italy, Netherlands, and Poland to name a few all collectively totaling 19 countries in Europe are banning GMO crops. Asia and Africa are excepting GMO crops more and more each year. One of the set-backs of gmo crops is the seeds. They have been nick named "terminator" seeds because you cannot re-plant the seeds from the crops grown. This is part of the cell manipulation and control mechanism of using GMO seeds for crops. It also was accepted as law that "owning" life as intellectual property was allowed. Therefore, farmer's using GMO seeds must purchase more each year without the access of perennials. There are hundreds of court cases between Monsanto and private Ma and Pop farms who have to spend thousands of dollars defending their businesses especially if they aren't using gmo seeds. These farms have to prove in court that their seeds aren't the property of Monsanto and that they do not owe them an annual royalty. Since the first GMO anti-biotic resistant tobacco plant was created in 1983, followed by the Flavor Savr tomato which was sold from 1994-1997 the list of GMO products has grown exponentially. Some of the foods that are known GMO crops are listed below.

GMO Crops List
meat, eggs, farmed fish, dairy, packaged foods, restaurant foods, corn products, soy products, sugar, canola oil, zucchini, papaya, wheat, rice, apples, tomatoes, alfalfa, sugar beets, yellow squash, cotton, potatoes, rapeseed, yeast, bananas, cassava, peas, aspartame and some honey.

To avoid GMO crops organic fruits and vegetables are the best way to go as well as growing organic fruits and veggies yourself is a great choice too to keep costs down. Also, looking for grass fed, non GMO grain fed, hormone/antibiotic free, and wild caught meats instead of farm raised is best, this includes fish. Tapping into your local organic farms as a co-op member is another great alternative and usually you can gain membership discounts for your organic produce. There really is a lot of community gardening programs popping up all over the U.S. if you want to learn hands on about gardening.

Powerful Daily Affirmations

Say in the morning and at night:

* I AM worthy of happiness and greatness
* I release what no longer serves me
* I AM healed and loved
* I forgive myself and others with unconditional love
* I AM deserving of my greatness

Food History
So, who the heck changed our food?

As I went deeper down the rabbit hole of educating myself about our food industry and habits, I began to ask the question, what did we eat before the industrial age in the U.S.? Me being a child of the era of industrialized fast food, I wondered what foods were indigenous to this land mass. And, who was responsible for cultivating it? This led me into a few interesting directions like, what did Native Indigenous peoples that had already been living in North America as early as 15,000 BC eat? All those centuries prior to the arrival of Christopher Columbus in 1492 (who never actually set foot in North America, but did land on various Caribbean islands as well as Central and South American coasts) and two, how did food change after the so-called arrival of Columbus and latter settlers? I was determined to find out who was behind the food changes in its beginning stages. Food and culture go hand and hand. So as the food changes, the culture changes, he who controls the food controls the people. Early North American foods varied according to the environment where each group lived. The Inuit that lived far north along the coast of the Arctic Ocean and in Alaska ate a lot of fish, seal meat and seaweed. As you could imagine, due to the bone chilling temperatures, growing and foraging for food may have proven to be difficult in such a climate. The Chinook and the Nez Perce people of the Pacific Northwest actually didn't farm and keep animals. They hunted and gathered their food. They mostly ate wild roots like wapato (a potato like vegetable) and huckleberries (akin to blueberries), and a lot of dried or roasted salmon that they caught in the Columbia River and other rivers that ran into Columbia. The Pueblo people of the Southwest (modern Arizona/New Mexico) had a diet of cactus fruit, pine nuts, rabbits and birds. Over in the Rocky Mountains and Great Plains the Sioux, Ute, Navajo and Cherokee people consumed a lot of

Mammoth until they died out, and a lot of buffalo meat that they dried and smoked to make jerky so they wouldn't waste any of the meat. They also ate pine nuts, and sunflower seeds that they gathered from trees in the area. Further east along the Mississippi and Missouri Rivers, people also ate a lot of fish and gathered nuts and berries. Along the Great Lakes, the Cree people ate fish with wild rice that they gathered in the wet lands. Over on the East Coast the Algonquin and the Iroquois people consumed venison (deer meat), fish, pigeon, turkey, rabbit, and sometimes bear. They also made bread out of acorn and sunflower seeds. The Cherokee people ate mainly corn, beans, and squash that they grew in their fields. The Cherokee also ate deer, rabbits, fish and turtles. The first people of North America to start farming planting and harvesting their own food were the Pueblo people. They learned how to farm corn, beans and squash from the Aztec people of Mexico around 2000 BC. But, they didn't really settle down and start farming for most of their food until about 100 AD. But, lets dig deeper and look at the African presence in America because; Africa is known to have cultivated crops over 12,000 years ago. One of the first recorded documented instances of Africans sailing and settling in North America were the Kemetians (renamed Egyptians) who were black people, led by King Ramses III, during the 19th dynasty in 1292 BC. In fact, Greek historian Herodotus wrote of the ancient Egyptian Pharaohs' great seafaring and navigational skills in 445 BC. Further concrete evidence, noted by Dr. Imhotep like the Egyptian artifacts found across North America from the Algonquin writings on the East Coast to findings in the Grand Canyon. In 1311 AD, another huge wave of African exploration to the new world was led by king Abubakari II, the ruler of the 14th century Mali Empire. The king sent out 200 ships of men, and 200 ships of trade materials, crops, animals, cloth and impeccable African knowledge of astronomy, religion and arts. So, now I bet you're wondering, what's my point? My point is, there's a connection between Indigenous peoples of North America, and African People's. Like many others, I once believed that the first Africans to arrive in North America were the "20 and odd" Africans who arrived as slaves in Jamestown VA., in 1619. So, what did they eat? They ate yams, watermelon, rice, eggplant, pigeon peas, maize (corn), barley, plantains, sorghum, coffee, teff, millet, black eye peas, and Kola nuts, whose extracts became an ingredient in Coca-Cola. Because of the cultivation of agriculture in Africa, they brought over an abundance of seeds and crops that they shared with the Indigenous peoples of North America that named the land mass "Turtle Island" before the conquerors came in and renamed it America. Because of all of the dehumanizing racism towards peoples of color and African descent, a lot of the contributions of Africans and their influence in North America is disguised or omitted for a plethora of reasons. But, we are in a time where the seals of secrecy have now been broken. There are also the interesting stories of African women who brought seeds over intertwined in their corn row braids. This is very significant because, there are a lot of crops indigenous to Africa that found their way to North America. The blending of Indigenous peoples in North America and African explorers created a mixing of culture, food, family, and spiritual practices. So, as we can see, very natural, unprocessed ways of eating was the normal behaviors. At that time people ate what was seasonally available in their regions including animal fare. If seeds brought from one region could not be cultivated in another region, it wasn't available. So, now that we have airplanes, ships, buses, and trucks, we can enjoy crops from other regions and countries without having to grow it where we are. Now, all countries can enjoy profiting from far beyond their borders thus, expanding their clientele market. However, it's a double edge sword because, a huge demand calls for big changes! The first change is that now, we have access to fruits and vegetables that originally would be "out of season" due to seasonal changes. But, now those gaps have been filled, but now we are eating outside the seasonal guidelines that connects us with the astrological planting cycles that correlate with the seasons. And with this movement came the need for extra charges to pay for fuel, trucks, airplanes, ships, packaging materials, international trading permits, warehouses, and trained workers just to name a few all come into play. So, with all of this going on, you almost have to guarantee your product for profit. Well, what does that look like? It looks like creating powerful herbicides and pesticides, and the adding of preservative's, and additives. Then, since it's all based on profit shelf life becomes the main issue instead of health. This huge turn of events mostly happened under our noses, and has landed us where we are now, trying to decipher this new industrial food age. This new food culture is not concerned about your healthy wellbeing, and it's obvious by the choices being made for us without our permission. Since fresh fruits and vegetables are the foods with the shortest shelf life, which spawned a downward spiral of large corporations hiring scientists to figure out a way to manipulate longer shelf life in fruits and veggies. That is what birthed the new GMO (genetically modified organisms) that we now call food. I have a whole chapter in this very book that breaks down GMO's and who's behind it. Once you start tampering with a food's natural ability to be, well *natural,* you have compromised that foods integrity. And, our bodies' intelligence does not recognize these new changes so out of this has birthed an influx of cancers, digestive problems, DNA damage, hormonal imbalances, diabetes, and sleep problems just to name a few. And, none of these companies asked us? Offered a vote? or gave us direct information on the effects on our bodies and our environment like they do with medications. Although cancer is up over

50% and moving towards 57% within twenty years, that means our current 1 in 2 people cancer diagnosis will increase. Child hood cancer is at an all-time high of 29% in the last 20 years and is increasing. Studies show that 1 in 330 children will be diagnosed with cancer by age 20. Lymphoblastic Leukemia is leading the way at a rate 21% in children. Cancer is also the leading cause of death in children in the U.S., it was second to accidents, but now cancer has surpassed that. Everyday 43 children are diagnosed with cancer and the average age is six. I'm no rocket scientist but, even I can clearly see the damage and health risks associated with the changes that have been made with our foods. It's certainly no coincidence that our health ailments are rising at a very scary and unbelievable rate and yet, no real concern or plan of action to address these concerns are being made. The bottom line is, we are whole beings, therefore, we need whole foods that are natural and in its original state, meaning the molecular structure is intact. There has never been a need to "create" over 300 varieties of apples. Corporations and their hired scientists are just looking for a reason to gain notoriety for "inventing" a new species of a plant or vegetable that is not needed outside of making a name for themselves. The old adage "If it's not broken, why fix it?" definitely applies here. Food is so different now, and as more lab crafted foods are introduced to the population, the further away we become from the true indigenous foods that our Ancestors' enjoyed with minimal to no health concerns. It is very clear that, the health of the people in North America took a wrong turn upon the integration of foods from cultures foreign to the original Indigenous peoples of North America.

The Food Label Drama
Legal lies for profit

Anyone who visit's a grocery store in this day in age, can bear witness to a plethora of food labels that make you "think" that you are purchasing a great healthy product that you can get the most nutrition out of for you and your family. However, there are some issues that need to be addressed concerning the truth and validity of such claims as "natural", "light", "low fat", and "sugar free" for example. The issue is that the definitions aren't all the way clear and, these labels are "made" to make you "believe" one thing while, the "legal" definitions are not what the average consumer thinks. Let's break down some of these definitions shall we?

All Natural
The FDA (Food and Drug Administration) had not as of yet established a formal definition. However, the USDA (United States Dept. of Agriculture) defines "all natural" as

having no artificial ingredients, no added color, minimally processed, and include a statement explaining its meaning. Well, that definition sounds very honest right? Well, what they aren't telling you is "all natural" also means using insects as a "natural" ingredient. And, they have the right to give it a different name so you won't recognize it in the ingredients list. Take for example, an ingredient called "confectioner's glaze" or "natural glaze". It's used in candy, vitamins, pills, tablets, capsules, chocolate, and waxed fresh fruit. But, what it really is, is Shellac? Shellac (commonly used as wood primer and varnish), is a resin which is secreted by the female Lac insect after it consumes bark. This insect is in the same family as the cochineal bug and lives on a variety of trees in Southeast Asia and Mexico. The raw resin is collected, heated, filtered, and mixed with an alcohol solution to create the food glaze. It is also used to hide odors in pills, and to make pills easier to swallow. Shellac has been known to cause allergic reactions in some individuals and, cause inflammation. But, where's the clear meaning of that on the packaging label?

Organic
The FDA says that organic means 95% is the minimal percentage to label a product as organic. Ok, seems harmless right? Well, what they're not telling you is this. By law, organic foods cannot contain synthetic fertilizers, industrial pesticides, antibiotics, growth hormones, or artificial food ingredients. But, the USDA maintains a list of "exempted" ingredients and once an ingredient gets on the list, it can be used for five years from the date of the exemption. The National Organic Standards Board, which is made up of 15 "non-governmental" experts. They decide on stuff like, should the use of an antibiotic called streptomycin be used on organic apples and organic pears?

Grain Fed
Grain fed implies exactly what it says. By definition, it means that in the first 6-

12 months an animal rather it's a cow, pig, or bison is fed grass, then afterwards fed grains. Well, what they're not telling you is the grains being used can be GMO grains and full of chemicals and the animals are still given antibiotics. Most grains given to animals as feed is industrialized chemical ridden grains. It is also interesting to note that, most farm animals are naturally drawn to eat grasses, and not grains. Grains have become the new age animal feed, thus changing the natural eating habits of farm animals, and an increase in E. coli in the gut of such animals. Animals being grain fed does not increase the vitamin content or quality of the meat, it's just that grains are the cheapest to produce for feed.

Low Fat
This means that the product contains less than 3 grams of fat per serving. Ok, seems simple right? Well, this applies to portion servings to "appear" at its healthiest amounts. Let's say for example, the portion size of a bowl of

cereal is ½ cup per serving at 3 grams of fat. Let's be realistic here! ½ cup of cereal is a child's portion! On average, an adult will easily consume at least 1 ½ cups of cereal per serving which is now sadly and easily 9 grams of fat. Not the idea you were thinking based on the package advertising. This stuff is tricky! That's just one reason why this book is needed.

Light/Lite

There's some very unclear business going on here! So, apparently the words "light" and "lite" can be used interchangeably. They both can mean 50% reduction in fat, calories, or sodium, even if the product says "light" without further explanation. What they aren't saying is that both words can also just mean that the product has a "light texture" or is "lite colored". Again, not what we expect based on the packaging label. They get a lot of sales with these particular labels from people who are dieting and "think" that they are purchasing a product that is healthier to support their weight loss needs, but with the sometimes lack of clarity, it may not.

Low Calorie/Calorie Free

Low calorie means no more than 40 calories (per serving), and calorie free means less than 5
calories. So, the issue with "low calorie" is if it contains a sugar substitute (sweet&low, splenda, or equal) for example, the 40 calories goes up. And, they can label a product "calorie free" and it still can have less than 5 calories. So again, based on the packages recommended serving size, which is always a small serving, let's say the serving is ½ cup of fluid, but that's barely enough to wet any adult's throat! On average an adult can consume 2 cups or more in one sitting. Now, you've consumed 160 "low calories" or close to 20 "calorie free" calories! Portion size with these products is a real issue that should be addressed because it is a tool they use to confuse and manipulate your eating and thinking.

Kosher/Parve

This label may only be used on labels of meat/poultry products that have been prepared under rabbinical super vision, in other words, it must be prayed over by a Jewish Rabbi. This has nothing to do with the product being organic, nor does it address antibiotics, chemicals, gmo grains, or the integrity of the meats quality. This is ONLY pertaining to religious prayer rites.

Halal/Zabiah

This label means that the meat/poultry must be handled according to Islamic Law under Islamic Authority. Again, this is prayer based and in some cases may pertain to the way the animal is killed. However, this has nothing to do with the product being organic, nor does it address antibiotics, chemicals, or gmo grain feed, or the integrity of the meat's quality. This is again, pertaining to religious prayer rites.

Chemical Free

Guess what? The word's "chemical free" by law cannot be printed on any packaging! Why? Because, due to all of these exempt lists, there's hardly ever a food product on the market that hasn't been exposed to some type of chemicals. So, don't expect to see this on any packaging any time soon, especially since we're unknowingly consuming a lot of chemicals/drugs "masquerading" as foods.

Did you know???
There's emotional sources of disease?

Allergies- denying self-power
Arthritis- feeling unloved, criticism, resentment
Bladder- anxiety, fear of letting go, being "pissed off"
Blood pressure-high: long standing emotional problems **low**: lack of love as a child, defeatism
Cancer- deep hurt, long standing resentment
Fibroids/Tumors/Cysts- nursing a hurt from a mate, blow to the women's ego

---

What the Heck are we eating?
Or, what's eating you?

So, as I've mentioned in previous chapters, we are eating a lot of chemicals and drugs. Let's get specific and go over some of these non-foods we're consuming. These are additives or preservatives created in a laboratory that is manmade and are often found to be carcinogenic (cancer causing) and able to affect your blood sugar, hormones, digestion, sleep, and mood. Also, know that ALL of these chemicals are listed as DRUGS or NEURO-TRANSMITTERS (brain chemicals that influence your mood and thoughts, facilitate communication between neurons in your brain) despite the food industries propaganda to convince you of otherwise.

MSG
Monosodium Glutamate is a flavor enhancer that's known widely as an addition to Chinese food, but that's actually added to thousands of the foods

you and your family regularly eat, especially if you are like most Americans and eat the majority of your food as processed or in restaurants. MSG is more than just a seasoning like salt and pepper, it actually enhances the flavor of foods, making processed meats and frozen dinners taste fresher and smell better, salad dressings tastier, and canned foods less tinny (unpleasant metallic taste). MSG is a toxic chemical that directly damages neurological tissue, as well as introducing a generalized endocrine disruption throughout the body known as "metabolic syndrome", the symptoms of which include hypertension, skin rashes, insulin resistance, elevated blood lipids, and/or elevated blood pressure. MSG is currently sold as a seasoning called "Accent". MSG is one of the worst additives on the market and is used in canned soups, crackers, meats, salad dressings, frozen dinners and much more! It's found in your child's school cafeteria, and amazingly, even in baby food and infant formula. In lab testing,

MSG administered to animals during the neonatal period resulted in reproductive dysfunction with both males and females. While MSG's benefits to the food industry are quite clear, this food additive could be slowly and silently doing major damage to your health.

Other Names for MSG: Hydrolyzed Vegetable Protein, Textured Vegetable Protein, Yeast Extract, Autolyzed Yeast, Gelatin, Textured Protein, Soy Protein Isolate, Whey Protein Isolate, Accent, anything hydrolyzed, anything protein.

High Fructose Corn Syrup
This is corn syrup that has been treated with enzymes to make it sweeter. It is about one and a half times sweeter than sugar. It's a mixture of fructose and dextrose. It does have calories, used in beverages, candy, frozen desserts, dairy drinks, canned fruits, processed meats, ice cream, and poultry. Again, it's great for industrial big business but, its toll on our health isn't looking good for us. For

starters, HFCS contains contaminants including toxic mercury that are not regulated or measured by the FDA. Some of the side effects of HFCS are enlarged heart, weight gain, obesity, increased risk of diabetes, hypertension, elevated "bad" cholesterol levels (LDL), liver damage, metabolic syndrome, immune system damage, speed-up aging process, mercury poisoning, insulin resistance, inflammation, leaky gut, and skin rashes.

Other Names for HFCS: Corn Syrup, Glucose Syrup, Tapioca/Fructose Syrup, Fruit Fructose, Crystalline Fructose, Corn Sugar, maltodextrin, corn sweetener, diglycerides, disaccharides, and Syrup Solids.

TBHQ
Tertiary Butyl hydroquinone, or TBHQ as it is more commonly referred to as, is in fact a chemical preservative which is a form of petroleum-derived butane (lighter fluid). It is used in foodstuffs to delay the onset of rancidness and greatly

extends the storage life of foods. This preservative is in so many products from food to shampoos and skin care products! It was put on the market after years of pushing by industrial food manufacturers to get it approved. TBHQ is either used alone or in combination with the preservative BHA (butylated hydroxyanisole) and/or BHT (butylatedhydroxytoluene). The FDA said that TBHQ must not exceed 0.02 percent of its oil and fat content. Death has occurred from the ingestion of as little as 5 grams. Ingestion of a single gram (a thirtieth of an ounce) has caused nausea, vomiting, ringing in the ears, delirium, a sense of suffocation, and collapse. Industrial workers exposed to the vapors suffered clouding of the eye lens. Application to the skin may cause allergic reactions. So, I'm willing to suggest that if you can't handle a chemical without gloves, you shouldn't be eating it! This toxic preservative is known mostly as TBHQ and doesn't have all of the tricky names as most other chemical additives and preservatives do.

FD and C Colors
Food, Drug, and Cosmetic Colors. A color additive is a term to describe any dye, pigment or other substance capable of coloring a food, drug, or cosmetic, on any part of the human body. In 1900, there were more than eighty dyes used to color food. There were no regulations and the same dye used to color clothes could also be used to color candy. In the 1950's children were made ill by certain coloring used in candy and popcorn. This led to the delisting FD and C Orange No. 1, Orange No. 2, and FD and C Red No. 32. Since that time, because of experimental evidence of possible harm, Red 1, Yellow 1, 2, 3, and 4 have also been delisted. Violet 1 was removed in 1973. In 1976, one of the most widely used of all colors, FD and C Red No. 2, was removed because it was found to cause tumors in rats. In 1976, Red No. 4 was banned for coloring maraschino cherries (its last use), and

carbon black (of all colors really?) was also banned, because both contain cancer-causing agents. Allura Red AC or Red No. 40 is a food dye that gets a lot of attention because, many American scientists feel that the safety of Red No. 40 is far from established because coincidentally, all of the testing was conducted by the manufacturer. Therefore, the dye should not have received a permanent safety rating. The Natural Cancer Institute reported that p-credine, a chemical used in the preparation of Red No. 40 was carcinogenic in animals. Rats given oral dosages of the coloring caused adverse reproductive effects. There are thousands of chemical lab made colors that are cancerous, poisonous, caustic, and DNA damaging. They play a game by creating a "temporary list". The provisional list permits colors to be used on a continuous provisional or interim, basis pending completion of studies to determine whether the colors should be permanently approved or terminated all together. When colors are on this list, they can postpone closing dates to extend the time it remains on the temporary list. What's really upsetting about this is that they are basically finding ways to utilize and test these chemicals on consumers like guinea pigs! But, what's even worse is, a huge portion of the population are not aware they are a part of a nationwide experiment! These corporations create "loop holes" to legally introduce chemicals into our food supply, even if it hasn't been tested! This clearly shows that our industrial food industry is "profit based" and not "pro-life" based as some of us recently thought.

Aspartame
Also known as NutraSweet/Equal, a compound prepared from aspartic acid and phenylalanine, with about two hundred times the sweetness of sugar. Aspartame is commonly found in "diet" foods. Whenever a product is labeled "sugar free", that usually means it has an artificial sweetener in place of sugar. While not all sugar-free products

contain aspartame, it is still one of the most popular sweeteners, making it widely available in a number of packaged goods. Some aspartame-containing products include: diet soda, reduced calorie fruit juice, gum, yogurt, sugarless candy and baked goods. Activist claim there's a link between aspartame and a multitude of ailments, including: cancer, seizures, headaches, depression, attention deficit disorder, dizziness, weight gain, birth defects, lupus, Alzheimer's disease, multiple sclerosis, blindness, decreased vision, tinnitus, severe tremors, abdominal pain, bloody stool, pain when swallowing, hyperactivity, and brain damage. This is actually a shortened list believe it or not! Aspartame also can trigger, mimic or cause the following illnesses: Chronic Fatigue Syndrome, Epstein-Barr, Post-Polio syndrome, Lyme disease, Grave's Disease, ALS, Epilepsy, Multiple Sclerosis, EMS, Hypothyroidism, Mercury sensitivity from Amalgam fillings, fibromyalgia, Lupus, John Hodgkin's disease, Lymphoma, and

Attention Deficit Disorder (ADD) There are 92 different health side effects associated with aspartame consumption. Aspartame has been on the market since 1974, and has been wreaking havoc ever since! And yet, the FDA and USDA chooses to turn their backs on numerous independent studies and the increase in all these illnesses over the last 40 years in the name of profit. What's even more interesting is, a lot of these chemicals and additives have been banned from most European Countries.

Artificial Substances
In foods, the term follows the standard meaning: a substance not duplicated in nature. A flavoring, for instance, may have all the natural ingredients but it must be called artificial if it has no counterpart in nature. One has to ask the question, if a product has all natural ingredients, but no counterpart in nature, then where are the "natural" ingredients from? Natural ingredients created in a laboratory setting, is NOT the definition of natural. Discrepancies

in the law like this, is what's so confusing to consumers.

Splenda
Or sucralose is an artificial sweetener made from sugar. It is about six hundred times sweeter than sugar but does not contain calories. The FDA approved sucralose in 1998, but it had been waiting for approval since 1987 in 15 food categories. It's used as a table top sweetener, in baked goods, fruit spreads, desserts, confections, and most of all diet drinks. Splenda has a long list of side effects like: gastrointestinal problems, migraines, seizers, dizziness, blurred vision, allergic reactions, blood sugar increases, weight gain, heart palpitations or fluttering, joint pains and aches, and neurological issues like anxiety, dizziness, spaced out sensation, and depression.

In conclusion, I want you to understand that our food industry is set up on the ability to make the highest profits by creating the lowest quality food products for the longest shelf life in order to fill their pockets. You must realize that in order to achieve this, food additives and preservatives comes into play. To retard food spoilage, chemicals' masquerading as food is a must for longer shelf life and profit! Some food products have more chemical content than actual food ingredients. This applies to your popular sports drinks, infant formulas, cereals, and juices that aren't 100% juice etc. It's not enough anymore to just eat something because it tastes good or even looks good. Did you know that a hamburger and fries from one of the popular fast food chains can be left out uncovered and NEVER decompose? Some private organizations have actually left this "fake food" out for 3 years or more! This lack of decomposition is what the chemicals and additives added to our foods are causing. Now, you eat this food, and it's like eating soft plastic or glue. This sludge's the blood on a molecular level eventually causing inflammation of the intestines, stomach, and your mood. These additives and preservatives are Neuro Transmitters, which are categorized as "drugs" by the FDA/USDA and has the ability to augment your brain function. These drugs historically came out of the terrible and unethical forced testing of the Jews by the Nazi's in Auschwitz, Germany led by Adolf Hitler in the concentration camps/extermination camps, from 1933-1945. Understand that mind control in the form of drugs added to food has been tested through experimentation years before it hits the market, rather the results of testing are made public or not. These drugs affect your spiritual sense, the way you think, your mood, and your ability to concentrate or exude deeper cognitive thinking, and mood. ADHD (attention-deficit/hyperactivity disorder) and ADD (attention deficit disorder) as well as depression are in fact by private studies connected to these drugs, as well as the ability to make one feel powerless and docile to forms of oppression. Interestingly enough, fluoride has a way of affecting one's mood to go along with things and not question them. The mixture of fear tactics in the media and nuero transmitter drugs in the food supply creates a control mechanism over us that we don't seem to notice. Do not allow yourself to be sold on the idea that our government would not do such a thing to the peoples of North America and abroad. We have to remember that the USA was in business with Hitler, made slavery a law, stole the whole continent of North America, created the Tuskegee Syphilis experiments, legalized segregation, Stole the continent of Africa, stole ancient writings and artifacts from other cultures, covered up true history and knowledge from the people, and now, we have a hard time accepting the truths right in front of our eyes. We are whole beings and so, we require whole foods to be healthy and happy! Anything else is a violation of our natural birth rites to be well and balanced.

Back to Nature's Basics

The path back to wellness

If you are on any medications or under a doctor's care, please consult with your doctor prior to using herbs beforehand, to learn about any possible contraindications

So, after all of that, the question is now what do I do now? But first, this is not about dieting; it's about lifestyle changes that you should be striving to do permanently. A diet is a means to achieve a certain goal in a short period of time like, losing ten pounds to get into an old dress etc. A lifestyle change is when you continue to eat healthy for the long term benefits for the entirety of your life. You have to take back your power as a consumer and become a food expert in your own right! It takes time and patience with yourself to change any habits or conditionings that you have been accustomed to for years of your life. Food is attached to our emotions and generational practices so, because of this, we see the same ailments and diseases running in a family. And, as we learn better, we do better. One can only start from where they are. So, if you're reading this, you are on a path of truth and need a change to become the healthiest and best version of yourself!

Getting Started with Basic Herbs 101

I know that earlier in the book, I went over some herbs to help with inflammation. However, I wanted to give you an expanded list of herbs to get you started, these are basic herbs that are the most easily accessible on the market. Herbs and food are our true medicine, always was and always will be. When we replace synthetic chemicalized medicine into our delicate body systems, we are opening ourselves up to a plethora of diseases and bodily malfunctions. Did you know that the oldest known book on herbs and their uses was written by the Kemetians (renamed Egypt by the Greeks) and the name Kemet is where they got the name "chemistry" from? "Kemistry", which is the study of the composition, properties, and reactions of matter, particularly at the level of atoms and molecules. The book is called The Papyrus Ebers, dates as early as 1550 BC, and is a 110-page medicine scroll, that was highly advanced for its time, and had an extensive set of pharmacopoeia. Kemetic medicine influenced later traditions, including the Greeks. The Greek Philosopher Homer in 800 BC wrote in the Odyssey; "in Egypt the men are more skilled in medicine than any of human kind". Hippocrates, (the "so called" father of medicine) wrote extensively about his observations of their medical practices. Herophilos, Erasistratus and later Galen all studied at the Temple of Amen Hotep, and acknowledged the contribution of ancient Egyptian Medicine to Greek Medicine. With that being said, the ancient teachings of Kemet still hold true, but none of it matters if you don't actually utilize and apply the information.

Forms of Herbs

Fresh- these are fresh picked herbs that can be boiled or dried to make a tea. Fresh herbs have the "shortest" shelf life if not dried.

Dried- these herbs have a longer shelf life of up to 2-3 years; you can either dry them by sitting them in direct sunlight, or by hanging them upside down with hemp or yarn string. It takes herbs dried this way anywhere from 2-7 days.

Liquid- this form of herbs is called a "tincture" or sometimes "herbal elixir" and this type has the longest shelf life of up to 5 or 6 years. This type of herbal mixture is usually in grain alcohol, which draws out the herbs medicinal powers, and stabilizes it while ceasing spoilage.

Herbal Dosages

Fresh Herbs- Adults: ½ ounce to 8oz of hot water. Children: ¼ ounce to 8oz of warm water.

Dried Herbs- Adults: 1 teaspoon to 8oz of hot water. Children: 1/3 teaspoon to 8oz warm water

Tincture- Adults: 30-40 drops or 1 dropper full under the tongue or mixed in water or juice. Children: 10-20 drops under tongue or mixed in water or juice

<u>Helpful "how to" Hints</u>

Boiling herbs

When boiling herbs always boil the water alone, turn off heat, then add herbs, cover and let steep for at least 20 minutes. If you allow tea to steep overnight it will be most potent the next day. This tea should be consumed within 2 days if refrigerated or 1 day if kept at room temperature. Try to avoid making tea in aluminum pots, if possible use metal or steel, as aluminum has been linked to brain malfunctions like dementia and Alzheimer's. You can also make "sun tea" by utilizing a gallon glass jug filled with water and your herbs, place outside in direct sunlight. Make sure to cap the bottle and, this process depending on the weather can take 2-9 hours.

Making Tinctures

To make your own "tinctures" typically 80-90 proof vodka is used, along with dried herbs. Use a small mason jar (16oz) and fill up 1/2 (stronger blends) or ¾ with herbs. Pour alcohol to the top of the jar and cover. *DO NOT* pack the herbs into the jar. Put the jar in a dark place in the back of a cabinet and let sit for a minimum of 6 weeks to up to six months for highest potency. *Don't forget to label your jars*

Herbs and their Benefits

Blood Purifiers: burdock root, pau di arco, yellow dock root, red clover, dandelion, sarsaparilla

Anti-Inflammatory: Alfalfa, bilberry, turmeric, cats claw, goldenseal, and feverfew

Female Reproductive/Hormonal Health: dong quai, cramp bark, vitex, false unicorn, wild yam, ladies' mantle, primrose, and red raspberry

Male Reproduction/Hormonal Health: saw palmetto, yohimbe, gotu kola, ginseng, maca root, and horny goat weed (hey I didn't name it! Ha ha ha)

Herbs Safe for Children: catnip, dandelion, marshmallow, rose hips, peppermint, chamomile, lavender, echinacea, fennel, and lemon balm

Herbs for Breast Feeding promotes/increases milk production:

chaste tree, chamomile, marshmallow, fennel, fenugreek, anise, oat straw, raspberry leaf

Herbs to dry up or decrease milk production: sage, peppermint, spearmint, chick weed, and black walnut.

Diabetes: ginseng, fenugreek, milk thistle, and cinnamon.

High Blood Pressure/Hypertension: chamomile, fennel, hawthorn berries, parsley, and rosemary.

Avoid Ephedra (ma haung) and licorice as both can elevate blood pressure

Depression: kava kava, st. john's wart, ginkgo baloba, and lemon balm.

A pinch of capsicum (red pepper) can be added to your herbal mixtures to "amplify" the other herbs. I would not recommend adding capsicum to children's herbal formulas.

You can mix and blend herbs together or use one herb at a time. Notice also that, a lot of these herbs are multipurpose as well, and that's what's so unique about herbs. Seldom do you see a pharmaceutical drug that is multipurpose in its usage like herbs. Herbs can be used internally or externally (used for aromatherapy). Allow your creativity and research to guide you in your herbal creations!

Did you know???

Herbs contain unique anti-oxidant, essential oils, vitamins, phyto-sterols, and many other plants derived nutrient substances, which help equip our body to fight against germs, toxins, and to boost immunity level. Herbs are, in fact, medicine in smaller dosages. Herbs and essential oils have in fact been found to have anti-inflammatory function by inhibiting the enzyme cyclooxygenase (COX), which mediates inflammatory cascade reaction inside the human body.

Did you know???

Aromatherapy oils and incense are an excellent way to heal your immediate surroundings and the body. Use this method when someone is bedridden or when meditating or to just uplift your space.

* **Myrrh**- nasal congestion, antiseptic
* **Frankincense**- nervous system, vasoconstrictor
* **Jasmine**- kidney, blood purifier, mineral stabilizer
* **Pine**- respiratory, digestion, organ cleanser, energy regulator, rejuvenator
* **Lavender**- cleanser of glands, pores and skin, mental tranquility
* **Rose\Sandalwood**- nerves, cleanser, pituitary gland, emotions

Shopping Guide/Replacement List
A help lists to guide you on your way!

As a rule, concerning food, anything that's bleached or "white" is devalued and lacks vitamin and mineral content which we need for our bodies to run at its highest efficiency. Anything that goes against that is laying the foundation for disease and disharmony to the body. Here is a list below of bleached foods that I recommend you remove from your diet immediately, with a recommended replacement list for those foods. Please remember that, your taste buds will need to readjust to the flavors of whole grains and foods high in valuable nutrients. The industrial fast food nation that we are now living in have programmed us to enjoy the taste of flavor enhancers and empty calories in the form of drugs(additives/preservatives), sugar, salt and grease, that are all chemicals masquerading as food. Allow yourself to adjust. Whole foods have a difference in texture and flavor so, do not expect to taste the same flavors, rather have patience with yourself and understand that you are in transition, and you take your new lifestyle change a day at a time. Introduce yourself to a new item weekly or set the pace that works best for you. The sooner you start, the better you will feel and look. Nobody ever said change is easy, but concerning your health, the short term and long term effects are beneficial and may even save your life! Do not underestimate the power of your bodies' ability to heal itself when you give it what it needs to build you up. Remember that the body renews itself and so, if you aren't at your best health, know that you can regenerate a healthier you within weeks of eating healthier. Below is a chart to show you the wonderful regeneration capabilities of your cells and organs. By feeding your body the right foods, you can enjoy a wealth of health within the first year!

Bleached "white" Foods: Bread, rice, pastries, refined flour, sugar, salt, cow's milk, and margarine.

Bleached "white" Food Replacement list: 100% whole wheat flour or 100% brown rice flour (gluten free) brown rice or wild rice, raw brown cane sugar/maple syrup, stevia, black strap molasses or honey, sea salt or Himalayan salt, almond, hemp or brown rice milk.

Organ and Cell Regeneration

Brain- 1 year (neurogenesis of the cerebral cortex)

Blood- 4 months (red blood cells 4 mos./white blood cells 1 year)

Skin- 1 month (epidermis/surface layer)

Lungs- 2-3 weeks (lung surface 2-3 weeks, alveoli (where exchange of oxygen and gases takes place, over a year)

Bones- 3 months (new bone cells 3 mos./ entire human skeleton 10 years)

DNA- 2 months (repairing of free radical damage)

Liver- 6 weeks (completely rebuilds itself in 6 weeks! And has the best regeneration rate of all the human organs)

Stomach- 5 days (epithelial-cell lining of the stomach rebuilds itself)

ALL twelve of your body systems; skeletal, integumentary, muscular, immune, lymphatic, cardiovascular, urinary, digestive, respiratory, nervous, endocrine, and reproductive, will benefit from healthier eating habits. Food/herbs in history were the original medicine, and we have been moved so far away from nature, that finding our way back has been challenging. My own trials and tribulations as a consumer caused me to ask questions and dig for the answers that weren't being offered on the surface level.

Salty Business

The story behind salt is very interesting because salt has been used by the Ancients for various reasons from seasoning foods, curing meats, to being used as a health aide to "re-mineralize" the body. Its uses were so vast that the trading of salt and herbs became big business. But, all salts are NOT created equal.

Common Table Salt (Sodium Chloride) is a poison. It affects the nerves, brain, muscles, bones, cells, glands, and bones. Table salt is also an irritant, dehydrates and oxidizes (rust) the tissues. This type of salt by example would be brands like Morton. But what is salt supposed to do? Salt regulates water content in the body and brain, blood pressure, promotes healthy blood sugar levels, promotes nutrient absorption in the intestine, and enzyme activation. Common table salt does not include all of the salts you need. The sodium chloride in table salt has been chemically cleaned and is in an unnatural form that your body doesn't recognize. So, the fact that common table salt is a "bleached" product we can clearly see why the body can't properly utilize it. It has been stripped of all nutrients, vitamins, and minerals and then, iodine is re-added afterwards. It's added to help prevent goiter. The thyroid is supported by iodine.

Salt Substitutes

Pink Himalayan Salt- This salt is 250 million years old! It has been exposed to high tectonic pressure surrounded by ice and snow high in the mountains. When observed under a microscope, this salt has a perfect crystalline structure. It is the highest grade of salt and contains all the natural elements that are found in your body (all 84) which are the elements that were found to be a part of the "primordial soup" in the beginning.

Sea Salt- Sea salt is very well known as another salt alternative to common table salt, however, seas salt does not offer the full range of mineral content like Himalayan salt, and, it offers minute amounts of minerals and even less iodine. It has the same basic nutritional content as table salt. It's not that much better, but over the past few years' sea salt has strongly been marketed as a great salt alternative, even though it's in the same neighborhood as table salt nutritionally. Stick with Himalayan Pink salt, it's not that expensive, and it can be found in health food stores and most, large food chain stores. Sometimes, you find some good deals by ordering online as well.

Tips to Live By

Eat Less CRAP:

C- carbonated drinks
R- refined sugar
A- artificial sweeteners & colors
P- processed foods

Eat more FOOD:

F- fruits & veggies
O- organic as often as possible
O- omega 3 fatty acids
D- drink plenty of water

Sugar Blues and other Truth's

Sugar along with salt is another food that was well traded in history. Did you know sugar was historically planted and harvested and refined by slaves? Then the sugar was used to buy slaves. The slaves were in turn sold by the pound, as individual livestock or as a group to buy rum made with white sugar. Then the rum was sold to buy slaves. This resulted in the sugar, slave, and rum trade. The most common sugar is white sugar (bleached) again all of the nutritional value has been stripped through the bleaching process. White sugar is refined carbohydrates and is technically classified as a drug. White sugar stresses the pancreas, kidneys, liver, and starves the brain of oxygen. On a psychological level, it affects memory, absent mindedness, and causes hyperactivity that leads to unacceptable behaviors. Most of us have experienced or witnessed the effects of sugar on children and how they begin "jumping off the walls" as the elder's would say, after consuming it. White sugar is extremely addictive and robs the body of vitamins and minerals. Avoid white sugar; it's devastating on the body.

Sugar Alternatives

Raw Cane Sugar- This is sugar care juice that has been evaporated. It is a light brown color due to it being minimally processed. However, it is processed! It is NOT the same as brown sugar, which is white sugar that has been sprayed with molasses. It does have a minimal amount of trace minerals but, nothing too significant. Sugar should be limited and used sparingly in your diet lifestyle.

Honey- This is a bee product. Honey has vitamins and nutrients in it because the bee's use it for food stores for the hive during the winter months when little to no nectar is available to them. If you suffer from pollen of ragweed allergies, honey may trigger a response. I don't recommend honey to sensitive individuals, and it should not be given to children under the age of 1 years old, due to their immature digestive system.

Stevia- This is a natural sweetener and sugar substitute extracted from the leaves of the stevia rebaudiana plant. It is 100 times sweeter than sugar. Stevia has no calories, but can have a slightly bitter flavor. It's a great sugar substitute for baking, however it does not caramelize. Some stevia products are more processed than others, look for brands that say "whole leaf" usually, it's minimally processed. This alternative is good for diabetics however, made sure it has no dextrose or maltodextrin in it, as it has no nutritional value, and can raise your blood sugar level. Stevia can be purchased in liquid or powder form.

Agave Nectar- This is syrup made from the agave tequiliana plant, and is mainly produced in Mexico. There's a lot of controversy around agave because it's not always clear if it has HFCS (high fructose corn syrup) in it. It's often promoted to diabetics because it has a lower glycemic index. It has a higher fructose content than any other sweetener, and higher than HFCS. Fructose is a major culprit in the rising incidence of type 2 diabetes and nonalcoholic fatty liver disease. I in recent years have discontinued the use because; I noticed that it caused inflammation in my joints. That for me is a huge indicator of HFCS being used.

Black Strap Molasses- This is a dark thick and sticky syrup that is produced when the sugar has been boiled out of the cane or beet juice. Whereas the toxic and unhealthy refined sugar is destined for our supermarket shelves, the highly nutritious molasses-which contains all the minerals and nutrients absorbed by the plant. Molasses is good for the hair, safe for diabetics, laxative qualities, rich in iron, high in calcium and magnesium. It is not as sweet as sugar. Use molasses in your cooking with caution, because molasses can overpower your baking with off-putting flavors. Until you're familiar with it, look for recipes that specifically call for black strap molasses.

Brown Rice Syrup- Brown rice syrup is made from brown rice that is soaked, spouted and cooked with a special enzyme that breaks the starch down into smaller, sweeter carbohydrate molecules. It's not as sweet as other sweeteners, and can have almost a caramel or butterscotch undertone. It is not recommended for baking. And there's an issue with arsenic being in some brands. I'm not a fan of brown rice syrup as, it seems to take more to sweeten tea and it augments the flavor of what you add it to.

Coconut/Date Sugar- Coconut sugar is made from the sap of the coconut tree. The sap is this evaporated to create sugar crystals. Coconut sugar can easily replace white sugar in almost all recipes without affecting the resulting flavor or texture of the food. Coconut sugar also has a lower glycemic index then many other sweeteners, so it doesn't spike blood sugar levels. Date sugar is made from dehydrated, ground dates and is used as you would brown sugar. The flavor is lightly sweet with butterscotch notes. Date sugar can be used in many baking recipes as a one-to-one replacement for white sugar or brown sugar. Make sure you use brands that are minimally processed and not refined or have added chemicals.

As the day's and years go by, the food industry will come up with more sugar substitutes due to the fact that people are coming into the realization that their eating habits are causing their ailments. The food industry will comply if the demand is high enough. The truth of the matter is; sugar is a specialty. Some people that are still living naturally may only experience sweet palate foods a few times a year. Same can be said for salt. But, what's interesting too is that bitters are the least palatal flavor of North America, with the exception of mustard greens being a food stable in most southern states.

Bread and Grains
The difference is….

All bread is not created equal! A lot of people are still consuming "white" or bleached bread. Most of us have a flavor palate accustomed to the taste of white bread. But, now that we know better, we must move towards 100% whole grain breads. The packaging of the bread must say 100% whole wheat of 100% whole grain. If it does not, then you are getting white bread, or white bread "sprayed" with food coloring to "appear" as wheat bread. I myself eat gluten free frozen bread that is organic made of potato starch or rice flour. Also, purchasing bread that is low in sugar and sodium is great too. The wheat that is being produced for consumption now is not the same wheat that our grandparent's or their parent's ate. This is the new gmo (genetically modified) wheat that our bodies' don't recognize as food, but as a foreign entity thus triggering our immune system. This is the reason why gluten sensitivity is on the rise! If you can find organic wheat bread, that is your best option. However, if you are a baker, baking your own from organic flour is as good as it gets because you know what's in it and you can fully trust it and not question any of the ingredients.

Quotes that stick!

Human beings can alter their lives by altering their attitudes of mind

- William James

All the world is full of suffering, it is also full of overcoming it
- Helen Keller

If is our duty as men and women to proceed as though the limits of our abilities do not exist
-Pierre Teilhard de Chardin

Live as you will have wished to have lived when you are dying
-Christian Furchegott Gellert

Oils and Fats
What's the big deal?

Healthy oils are always a big deal because; the body needs healthy oils for a number of reasons from joint lubrication to healthy skin. However, the wrong oils can wreak havoc on the body by accumulating and depositing in organs and blood vessels etc. Lard (pork or beef fat), corn oil, canola oil, and rapeseed oil are amongst the worst oils you can use because they are not water soluble (dissolves in water) and the body can't properly flush out the excess oils after digestion. And, these oils are usually genetically modified, highly acidic and clogging such as saturated fats/trans fats. What you want in your diet is "unsaturated fats". It's time we embrace the healthy oils/fats.

Extra Virgin Olive Oil- This oil is full of oleic acid (a monounsaturated, omega-9 fatty acid) that benefits the balance of total cholesterol, LDL and HDL cholesterol in the body. EVOO (extra virgin olive oil) has also been proven to have anti-inflammation properties. This oil has been used for centuries. However, EVOO has its own set of cooking rules. It's stable for salad dressings, drizzled over steamed veggies, soups, breads, and light sautéing. EVOO is not good for high heat recipes. Olive oil loses its nutrients and can become unhealthy if heated over 275 degrees. It's NOT the right oil for frying foods.

Coconut Oil- In recent years, coconut oil has made its way to the fore front. Its unique combination of fatty acids can have profound effects on health. This includes fat loss, and better brain function. Coconut oil is in fact, a saturated fat, and one of the richest natural sources known to man, with almost 90% of the fatty acids in it being saturated. Additionally, coconut oil doesn't contain your average run-of-the-mill "artery clogging" saturated fats like you would find in cheese or meats. Instead of long chain triglycerides (fatty acids) it has medium chained triglycerides which are metabolized differently than long chained. They go straight to the liver from the digestive tract, where they are used as quick source energy or turned into "ketone bodies" which can have therapeutic effects on brain disorders like epilepsy and Alzheimer's. It's also best for low heat to medium cooking. It's a super food at best!

Palm Oil- This oil is an orange reddish oil from the African oil palm Elaeis guineensis. Palm oil has a distinct flavor that the North American palate may need to get used too. Palm oil is full of carotenoids, sterols, vitamin E, and powerful antioxidants like phenolic acids and flavonoids. This oil is great for frying foods up to 450 degrees. It takes some getting used to but know that 40% of the people in the world use palm oil, it's just rarely known in America.

Avocado oil- This oil is another rich source of Oleic Acid (healthy fat) that puts it on the map as having some wonderful qualities similar to olive oil except avocado oil can be used for high heat frying up to 520 degrees! And, it has a great light tasting flavor. This oil can help keep hormones in balance, heart health, good source of vitamin E, improves digestion, weight loss, strengthens skin, grows hair fuller/faster, reduces inflammation, itching, and accelerates wound healing. I'm a fan of this oil too because it's good for so much!

Butters/Margarine- Real butter made from milk is said to be the healthiest butter however, unpasteurized (unprocessed) butter is said to be even better! Margarine can either be vegetable shortening or a mixture of dairy and vegetable oils blended together. As far as the body is concerned, animal fats do not operate well in the body, and animal fats clog arteries the fastest! These oils are not water soluble and are fat soluble meaning their not so easily flushed out of the system. Margarine is a fully processed product usually full of soybean oil that is highly acidic and gmo. I'm not a fan of either and, I would look for vegan brands of butter "substitutes" that are coconut or olive oil based.

Tips for Success!

* Join a health food co-op
* Form a buddy system or support group
* Take food preparation classes
* Meditate on a healthier you
* dance, sing, and play!
* Sit in nature often
* Be the change you want to see
* Keep a journal to write out your feelings and emotions, over time you can go back and see your growth.

Know Your Resources!

There's tons of resources out there to assist you on your journey to wellness. Here's a list of ideas to get you on your way!

*Library: The library offers a large selection of FREE books and DVD's, from cookbooks to magazines that assist you with recipes, exercises, and motivation.

*Internet: You can "google" and search for recipes, how to guides, as well as utilize YouTube for the FREE helpful cooking tutorials and exercise videos.

*Local Classes: Your local area may offer classes through the clinics, hospitals, Dr. offices, chiropractic offices, libraries, and even your local fire station. If not, start requesting them. Some are free and some are very inexpensive.

*Ask Around: Word to mouth is a strong way to find what you seek! Go to people you consider healthy and ask them what they know and what resources can they share with you.

The Meaty Melt Down

There will always be controversy around if we should consume meats or not. As a human race we have consumed both over generations of time. However, studies consistently show that plant based diets are the best. The absence of artery clogging fats, unprocessed foods, whole grains, fresh fruits and vegetables, and clean water has shown lower accounts of developing cancers, hypertension, and HBP, as well as potentially healing and preventing a long list of ailments. Our Ancestors consumed larger portions of vegetables and grains, with meat being the smallest portion in their diet. We have to be clear about where this culture of large meat consumption comes from. Our body does need protein to survive however; meat protein is not the best source, but a source. Historically, Europeans who lived in the Caucus Mountains in cold and damp environments did not have the best access to fruits and vegetables like those living in warmer climates, like the

Africans' or the Asians for example. Coming out that history, it only makes since that the Europeans who set the tone in eating meat as a regular dietary staple would put meat at the forefront. Culturally, fruits and vegetables were secondary in their diet. Meat as a dietary supplement is based on European culture and NOT medical reasons. There's no original writings out of European culture that predates Egypt's (Kemet) writings about herbs and health. And, as a matter of fact, Hong Kong carries the record for the longest life longevity on earth currently! And, they consume more veggies and fruits more than meat. The numbers don't lie, but our current eating culture will, especially when it's built on profit, and not truth and concern for human life, nature life, or tomorrow's environment. I am not here to push a vegan or vegetarian lifestyle on you, but rather to show you our programming and how it has affected our personal lives as well as our loved ones. If meat consumption is the choice you choose, my advice would be to buy organic "grass fed" meats and avoid beef because it takes the longest to digest, and pork, because it carries the most parasites of all the meats. Poultry and fish baked, grilled or boiled is much better than fried. Consider eating more veggies and grains and a small cut of meat. But, if you want to transition to eating a vegan or vegetarian diet for a lifestyle change, then you can start with a day or two a week, if so, read on!

Meat Substitutes

For starter's I am not a huge fan of meat substitutes, but for those transitioning, they are a "temporary" food to get you started. I am not a fan of processed foods and most meat substitutes are processed. I love vegetables, and since I have been a vegan since 1998, and I have learned that the rich offerings of grains, fruits, and vegetables reign supreme in that, I'm still discovering and creating wonderful recipes that are fulfilling and no! I'm never starving or feeling hungry. As a matter of fact, one time, at a checkup, my then doctor assumed that because I was vegan, my iron was low, but lo and behold it was within normal range and, he also assumed my protein was low and it was too high! Lol…. I actually had to cut back on my plant protein!

Soy- Soy initially was not supposed to be consumed by humans, as it was to be used for animal feed. Soy is usually processed into blocks, crumbles, sauces, and a plethora of meatless products. It's the easiest meat substitute to find at any food store and it comes in an array of culinary choices. However, soy is high in estrogen, and soy is in a lot of food products that aren't considered vegan or vegetarian that has soy isolate, or soy protein as an ingredient or filler. When too much soy is consumed, it can affect the hormones by causing you to have excessive amounts of estrogen in your body which can cause cancers and inflammation. There is a "quite" epidemic of young boys' and men growing excessive breast tissue due to excess estrogen in their bodies, and with the issue of all cancers on the rise at 52%, we need all the help we can get.

Seitan (wheat meat) - Seitan is derived from the protein portion of wheat. Seitan is also another word for "wheat gluten". So, this is a wheat product, and if you eat gluten-free like me, then this may not be for you. Seitan has a meaty texture and can be used in place of chicken and beef recipes. It works well in stews, stir-fry's, pasta's, and fajitas!

Mushrooms- Mushrooms take the flavor with ease and provide a tender and hearty texture, and good protein to curve cravings. Mushrooms come in a huge variety of sizes and textures from buttery soft, to beefy tough. You can sauté or bake them for pizzas, sandwiches, and wraps. They can also be fried crisp and used in veggie BLT's and breakfast dishes! Try to get organic mushrooms as often as possible.

Jackfruit- This is one of the new kids on the block in vegan/vegetarian eating. Jackfruit is a fibrous miracle fruit from India that offers a shredded, tender consistency to give a number of dishes a great texture. This fruit is so versatile that you can make "mock" dishes like barbeque pulled pork, chicken salad, Philly cheese steak, taco's, tuna melt's, crab cakes, and sloppy Joe's! Nature's offerings are amazing if you are willing to learn.

Beans/Legumes- There are so many kinds of beans that, one could eat a different variety every day of the year. Legumes are nutritional power houses that deliver tons of fiber and protein for pennies on the dollar. Beans can be used in soups, tacos, and to make bean patties' for burger substitutes'. I prefer dried beans, and they should be soaked overnight before cooking to help rehydrate them and to speed up cooking time. I love beans cooked down in a crock pot, with a nice hunk of cornbread!

There are some brand's that sell organic beans in a can for quicker options.

Did you know???

Foods give off vibrations? Scientifically, fruits, veggies, and whole grains have the highest vibration because of the sun's energy charge locked inside. These foods are also the most healing because of it. The lowest vibrational foods are meat, processed foods, fast foods, and any foods that have been bleached and devitalized. These foods are full of sugar, dyes, chemicals, and empty calories that promote disease in the body. Now, you can see why the high vibrational foods are necessary when fasting and cleansing.

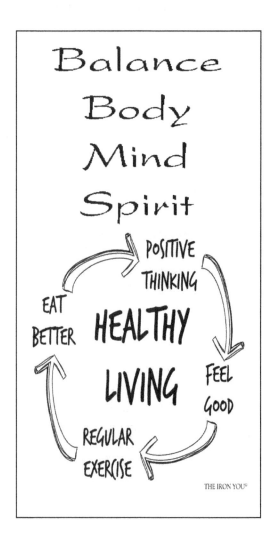

Balance
Body
Mind
Spirit

POSITIVE
THINKING

EAT
BETTER HEALTHY

LIVING

FEEL
GOOD

REGULAR
EXERCISE

THE IRON YOU©

106

The Spices of Life

When it comes to the flavor of food, nothing enhances like herbs or "seasoning". Most people dislike the taste of foods without it. It's very difficult to consume meat products without seasoning, so ultimately using seasonings on veggies also takes the flavors to the next level. I am a fan of growing your own seasonings. They are super easy to grow in small pots in your window sills. They grow pretty fast and you can dry them and store them in your own creative containers. Herbs like oregano, parsley, cilantro, sage, tarragon, basil, rosemary, and bay leaves are easiest to grow. Of course the other alternative is to buy your herbs. There's, tons of brands out there that offer a plethora of blends, some with salt and some salt free. Whenever possible, purchase the organic brands, and if it contains salt, make sure it isn't white table salt but rather Himalayan pink salt or sea salt. The issue with buying prepackaged bulk herbs is that they can contain insect fragments that are hard to detect with the naked eye. Keep reading and I will discuss that later in this book.

What is Fasting???

There are various types of fasts like water, juicing, wheatgrass, raw foods, and religious. And the purpose is to purge and allow your body, mind and spirit to release toxins, and emotional baggage. You can fast for one day, weeks or do it seasonally. It's also a good practice to fast one day out of the week. In nature, when animals are not feeling well they fast on water or sometimes they eat certain grasses and herbs. As humans, we should do the same. If you start to feel sluggish and fatigued on an ongoing basis, perhaps it's time for a fast to reboot and reset your body. Consult with a physician and do your research before you choose any fasting method especially if you're on any medications.

Think Before You Drink!

Is Juice Created Equal?

No! It is not. Most juice "drinks" is being passed off as real juice products, yielding more chemicals and food coloring than actual juice. Some of these products are riddled with HFCS (high fructose corn syrup) as well as additives, and preservatives. Look for juice labels that say 100% juice, no HFCS, and preferably no added sugar. There are a lot of brands that say anywhere from 0% juice to 50% juice, and the rest is water and dyes and chemicals. And some brands offer more vitamin C than juice! Go for organic and try juicing yourself whenever you can. You will definitely notice a price difference in food the better the quality, however start a small garden or look for local organic farms and natural food stores in your community that way, you get your veggies super fresh when it's nutrient content is at its highest. Some local farms offer membership packages, where you can receive discounts and special access before the regular public. Another plus is developing a personal relationship with the people that grow your food. And, in most cases the opportunity to volunteer and learn to farm for FREE!!! Imagine that???

Did you know???

In the early years of the twentieth century, hamburgers had a bad reputation. According to historian David Gerard Hogan, the hamburger was "a food for the poor", tainted and unsafe to eat.

French Fries are cancer causing cooked trans fatty acid! It is mostly grease then potatoes! 50 grams or more of fat per serving and its indigestible. French fries are ranked one of the worst chemicalized GMO foods on the market!

Alternative: Buy sweet potatoes, leave the skin on, cut into French fries and bake in the oven until golden brown.

The Diary of Dairy

Dairy takes on a different definition depending on who you're talking too. But the media has always sold dairy as a wholesome healthy product that's good for your muscles and bones. But, the truth is, most people of African descent are lactose intolerant, another percentage has a milk allergy, and another portion is allergic all together. Dairy is also a processed food. Foods like cheese, yogurt, butter, and ice cream are the most commonly consumed dairy products. Dairy products have consistently tested positive for hormones, antibiotics, GMO's and pesticides, over the past 10 years, as well as some of them being known carcinogens' (cancer causing). To top that off, dairy carries a lot of pus from the inflammation of over milked teats (mastitis). Did you know that humans are the only species on the planet that consumes the milk of another species? And only humans continue to consume milk well into adulthood. But, don't worry, there's a solution.

Soy Milk- This is the most popular on the market, but not the best. Soy is very high in estrogen, but it does have a heavy milky consistency like vitamin D milk. It does work well for recipes that call for milk, and works well as a milkshake base. You can also find soy ice cream and yogurt as well. Look for organic.

Almond Milk- This versatile nut milk that can also be used as a dairy substitute, as well it also offers calcium and protein. Look for organic.

Coconut Milk- Coconut is a powerful antioxidant packed fruit! So, naturally its milk is rich too! It's great for baking as well but, use the unsweetened kind as, coconut can give off its own slightly sweet flavor. It's great as a fruit smoothie base, and yogurt. Again, look for organic.

Rice Milk- This milk is the lightest and most translucent of all the alternative milks. Look for brown rice milk; otherwise it's made from white (bleached) rice. This milk is the "skim milk" of the vegan world. If you like lighter milk, this one's for you. It's not the best for cooking and baking, but it can make a decent smoothie base and the ice cream is tasty, smooth and melts a bit faster.

These are the basic milk and dairy substitutes that can easily be found or homemade. The best benefits of dairy are to consume it raw and unpasteurized. You would then have to find a local farm that can safely handle and sell raw dairy products like milk, cheese, yogurt, and cream. It has a much shorter shelf life, which is frowned upon by industrial big business. And you must always do your research and consult with your physician before consuming raw unpasteurized dairy products. And never give raw unpasteurized dairy to infants or children.

Did you know???

Soda is basically liquid chemicals, sugar,
artificial dyes, artificial flavoring, and
carbonated water that dehydrates you.
And, not to mention the empty calories that
affects your blood sugar and triggers excess
weight gain.

Alternative: look for naturally brewed
ginger beers, fruit juices, and root beers
with real fruit and no artificial or chemical
ingredients. You can find this at your local
health food stores or at regular food chain's
that offer a health food "section".

Crazy but legal food facts

Have we gone mad???

Mass food production comes with a lot of responsibilities because the aim is profit at your expense. With that, comes the need to cover themselves legally in case anything from allergic reactions to death occurs from people consuming their products. But, in between are some allowances concerning our food that you may not be so happy to know. Welcome to yet another dark side of the industrial food age. Understand that, industrial food plants attract a lot of uncontrollable bugs and rodents etc. so legally, they had to include them.

Legally…...

*Peanut butter can contain 1 or more rodent hairs per 100 grams (7/8 of a cup)
*Canned mushrooms must have over 20 maggots per 100 grams and proportionate liquid to sue.
*Ground oregano must have less than 1250 bug fragments per 10 grams.

*Sesame seeds can have 5% or more insect fragments by weight.
* Canned tomatoes can have 10 or more fly eggs 500 grams (1.10 lbs.).
*Tomato juice can have 10 or more fly eggs per 100 grams.
*Wheat bread can have 1 or more rodent hairs per 50 grams.
*Canned beets can contain 5% or more of dry rotted pieces
*Mites in your frozen broccoli
*Maggots in your brined or Maraschino cherries
*Parasitic cyst in your fresh water herring
*Mildew in your canned greens
*Mold in your apricot, peach, and pear nectars.
*Worms and mold in your canned and frozen peaches.
*Larvae in your canned or frozen spinach
*Rodent "pellets" in your wheat

These food legalities can go on and on! I just wanted to point out a few really disgusting one's to show you what you are eating. I prefer fresh over frozen or canned goods, because that way I can bypass a lot of the above listed issues. It's time to get back to natural living and eating again! When you know better, you do better! Happy Healing! For more info on the Author and Bookings for classes, lectures, or retreats Zema Love Fire can be reached at Zemalovefire@gmail.com

"The real magic is knowing that you deserve the best, and creating a lifestyle that supports that by you choosing to develop a "be the best version of yourself philosophy" can only turn into a better and fuller quality life"

---Zema Love Fire

Did you know???

Your body has a digestive cycle and if you eat in accordance with it, you will see improvements in your energy, bowel movements, sleep patterns and overall wellbeing.

Breakfast 5am-11am- Light foods as you are "breaking a fast after resting" fruits, smoothies, oatmeal, or teas

Midday 12pm-4pm Lunch/early dinner – This is the time when the sun is at its strongest point for the best digestion. Eat your heaviest meals and foods of the day during this time span.

Late day 5pm-8pm Dinner- At sunset, your body starts to go into rest mode to sleep and recuperate for the next day. So, another light meal like a salad, soup or smoothie is ideal because otherwise heavy foods will ferment and poison the system

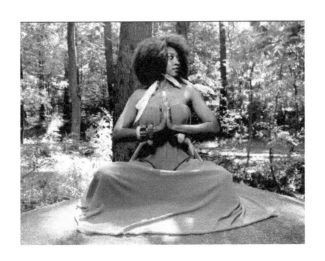

About The Author

Zema Love Fire is a Natural Living Advocate, Food Researcher, Vegan Chef, Author, Reiki Master, Vibrational Therapist, Rites of Passage Facilitator, Teacher, Jazz Fusion Artist, and Creative Muse. Born in Savannah, Ga. As a former asthma sufferer who nearly died from breathing complications as a child, suffering from painful urinary tract infections, eczema, and inflammation, she knew early on that something wasn't right. Zema realized that there was a connection between food and health. Her mission became questioning everything she put in her mouth. In 1998 Zema chose a vegan lifestyle after her first year of researching food and the new industrial foods which included an abundance of chemical ridden, denatured, cancerous, and disease inducing foods. The rabbit hole runs very deep concerning our food, and this guide will take you on a ride down that hole, offering shocking but true information about what we are eating, and what's eating you! For more info on the Author and Bookings for classes, lectures, or retreats Zema Love Fire can be reached at the following:

Website: TheNewFoodCulture.Com
Email:zemalovefire@gmail.com
Facebook: Zema Love Fire
Twitter: FireZema
Instagram: Zema Love Fire
Periscope: FireZema

Special Thanks….

Hair Stylist/Kim Savage

Photographer: Hakim Wilson
 photobrothersmedia.com

Set Assistant: KemKemJ
Natural Kemistree

Bob Johnson: Director of Juneteenth
Atlanta Parade & Music Festival
Juneteenthatl.com

www.thenewfoodculture.com

Ordering information

Quantity sales: Special discounts are available on quantity purchases by corporations, associations, and others. For details, contact the publisher at the address above.

Orders by U.S. trade bookstores and wholesalers:
Please contact The Love Fire Group
(470) 242-1659